Certified or CertiFRAUD?

Assessing the Professional Competency of Your Personal Trainer- Who's Minding Your Store?

Anne Larson, EdD

ISBN: 1-4699-5468-0
ISBN-13: 9781469954684

Forward

One bad haircut and you don't return to that stylist. One sloppy hedge trim and you find a new lawn service. One masseuse with questionable behavior and you sprint away without looking back. One server with a poor attitude and you swear off the restaurant.

Ineffective training sessions with an incompetent personal trainer – you sign up for additional sessions.

Ugh!

With perfect intent you seek a professional partner to help guide your fitness journey. But the process can be daunting, perhaps intimidating, given the perception you possess limited capacity to make a sound choice. So you rely on opinions of others or agree to work with whomever your gym assigns. Unfortunately, this may or may not be in your best interest. For like any service-based profession, some are capable, others are not.

Please know that I am on your side. While there is no excuse for incompetency it's you who suffers too, for their underachievement leads to your underachievement!

The good news – good trainers exist. The other good news – even without a background in exercise science you can come to understand principles that underlie effective personal training. With but a bit of effort you can learn to discern the good from the waste of time, the certified from the certiFRAUD.

I hope you find what follows useful—after all, you are the only one of you, you get—and wish you the best along your path to optimal well-being. To your health!

"Any weight more than 10 pounds is for men."
"Your heart rate should be like way over 200."
"I can make your arms look like Angelina Jolie's."

Overheard comments made by personal trainers to their clients

Physical activity participation can hold THE key to lifelong wellness and independence—a fact that isn't lost on most.

But doing trumps knowing, and sadly at no other time in history has our nation been as fat and underactive as now. Two-thirds of adults carry unhealthy weight and fail to engage in the minimum recommended amount of physical activity. Left unchecked, the likely consequence is a myriad of physical, cognitive, and emotional issues that can sorely impact quality of life and ultimately result in premature death.

Yet, in spite of a sputtering economy, more people than ever belong to a fitness facility. In 2011, over 50 million people belonged to one of about 30,000 fitness facilities across the country, and 6.5 million use a personal trainer.

So what gives?

In a perfect exercise world, doing necessarily follows knowing. We know we need to exercise; therefore we exercise. Simple. But unfortunately it's not always so simple to take the first step, then the next, and then do it all again the next day.

Toward the intent to develop and sustain a regular physical activity habit, we join a gym. And to enhance our motivation to exercise, many of us hire a personal trainer. You may well be one of the existing 50 million gym members and/or 6.5 million who use a personal trainer. For good reason, gym members are more physically fit than non-gym members, and personal trainers can profoundly influence our motivation to exercise and adhere to a regular habit of participation.

But maybe you are one of the 60 percent of gym members who don't use their membership. Or maybe your personal trainer doesn't possess the professional capacity to guide your health-related fitness.

Using a personal trainer can be an invaluable asset. It can influence our motivation to sustain an activity habit and help us reap the health-protective benefits that participation can yield. But just how **competent** is your trainer? Is he/she able to deliver the necessary goods to foster your gym achievements? Or is he/she training you to underachieve?

Hopefully the comments made by trainers and repeated above sound outrageous to you in your experience with a trainer. Sadly, however, they may not be if your own trainer lacks the professional competency to induce your health-related wellness.

But how can you tell?

Selecting a trainer with whom to work is a significant decision that ought to be considered with great care. A point that can't be stressed enough—*considered with great care*! After all, you will be regularly spending chunks of time with him/her in a context that is both physically and emotionally challenging. Mostly, though, it's a critical decision for what is at stake for you—your health-related well-being. In no way can you afford to entrust your well-being to an incompetent fitness professional.

Being an informed consumer is the variable that can ensure the trainer you choose can deliver results.

The purpose of this book is to illustrate the qualities and competencies that distinguish a quality trainer from an ineffective one. Included is a systematic protocol you can use to aid your selection of a trainer and/or assess the quality of the one with whom you are currently working. The content is intended to inform your ability to assess a trainer's professional competency so you are empowered to ensure their ability to guide your achievement.

The biggest reason to make a thorough assessment of your trainer? The stakes are too high to work with a trainer who does not possess the professional aptitude or attitude to deliver results.

Is Your Trainer Training You to Underachieve?

Personal trainers are not born. They are created by engaging in formal academic coursework that fosters the acquisition of a broad range of content knowledge, experiencing multiple forms of physical activity, gaining an appreciation of the human experience related to physical activity, and becoming astute at motivation related to physical activity participation. Nor are personal trainers effective simply because they are good conversationalists, or are nice, or have a nice physique, or have time available to work with you.

Personal training is a profession with its own proprietary knowledge base, set of skills required for effectiveness, and established protocol to guide service delivery. It would be a relief to be assured that all personal trainers are adequately prepared to engage in their work, but like other service professions, some trainers are good and some are not.

Considering the stakes, we owe it to ourselves to make sure that the personal trainer in which we entrust our health-related well-being, and pocketbook!, possess the aptitude and attitude to induce benefit. While hesitant to say 'wasted time' this is what you risk if your trainer does not possess the competency to appropriately foster your health-related achievement. More than wasted time though, its wasted opportunity for enhancing your well being.

But, you say, my trainer is "certified." Doesn't that mean he/she is qualified?

Unfortunately, a resounding NO!

"Certification" in and of itself does not at all guarantee competency. There are hundreds of organizations in the United States that "certify" personal trainers, but only a very small percentage of these are considered to be viable preparation; or deemed reputable by being third-party accredited by the National Commission for Certifying Agencies (NCCA). (Please refer to Appendix A for a list of NCCA-accredited organizations.)

Many of the rest will "certify" a trainer by completing an on-line seminar or attending a weekend preparation program. This type of "certification" isn't worth even the value of the paper document acknowledging one's distinction as a trainer. Certification can unfortunately be "certifraud!" by developing trainers who sadly are <u>well-intended but mis-informed</u>.

Trainers who are well-intended/mis-informed often have personalities that make them very popular at gyms—they are friendly, outgoing, always pleasant, always smiling. But for how it relates to fostering your achievement at the gym, there needs to be substance along with the smile for you to avoid underachievement. Why?

<u>A primary factor that determines the difference between someone who is an expert physical activity professional from one who is merely an effective physical activity professional is content knowledge</u>.

That is, the more one knows about the components of health-related fitness, the content, the more likely it is that learning, i.e., improved health-related fitness, will occur. Working with a well-informed trainer is critical to your gym achievement. Of course, a combination of the two is optimal; a fitness professional who possesses strong content knowledge and maintains a pleasant demeanor.

Being a well-intended but mis-informed or under-informed fitness professional is simply not good enough. Don't ever compromise your health-related well being by continuing to work with (and pay!) a trainer who does not possess the attitude or aptitude to be accountable to your health-related achievement. His or her underachievement should not yield your underachievement.

So, how can you be sure that your trainer possesses the professional capacity, the aptitude, and the attitude to foster your gym achievement?

What follows are points to consider when assessing the professional competency of a trainer. After all—and this is a critical point—you DO have a choice as to whom you employ.

First, if you are not already, you need to become an informed consumer. Being an informed consumer entails two aspects: a) understanding the basic principles of achievement-oriented health-related fitness and b) using a structured protocol to inform your decision about hiring or continuing to employ a trainer.

1. Health-Related Fitness 101: What We Need To Know

Physical activity participation is good, why? It can be health-protective.

The beginning is always the best place to start, and the beginning that seems to make the most sense here is a primer that outlines the good that can be gained through physical activity participation. I am certain that the notion "physical activity is good for us" is not lost on the vast majority if not everyone reading this. Yet, confounding paradoxes exist about our relationship to physical activity that make it apparent that simply believing in the notion hasn't served us well. Knowing and doing seem to be two separate things, and even for those who are active, many seem to be missing the mark when it comes to doing what is needed to yield benefit.

Achievement-Oriented Health-Related Fitness is an approach to physical activity participation whereby one engages according to what is required to yield health protection. While engaging in some physical activity is more healthful than engaging in no physical activity, the *type* of activity and *manner* in which it is done has to be considered so the five components of health-related fitness—cardiovascular strength, muscular strength and endurance, flexibility, and body composition—are impacted.

What follows is a description of the protocol required to stimulate achievement (benefit) in each component. To realize health protection through activity participation we need to abide by the parameters that dictate beneficial engagement. The intent is to convey accurate, key information about achieving within each component. This is essential content knowledge toward determining if your routine will in fact yield results as well as the professional competency of your trainer or potential trainer.

But before we move forward, a few misconceptions need to be addressed:

First, there is a difference between the concepts of "performance-related fitness" and "health-related fitness." Performance-related fitness can encompass elements of sports-related physical activity. Health-related fitness encompasses that of physical activity that yields health protection. Being able to proficiently throw a ball, a sports-related measure of performance, in and of itself will not yield any health-related benefit. Throwing a ball as part of an activity that fosters cardiovascular or muscular strength, though, can yield health-related benefit. Considering the importance of sustaining our well-being, that which pertains to achieving health-related fitness is the underlying premise of this book.

Second, and related to the first point, the realm of physical activity is not an exclusive, secret society meant only for the athletically gifted. Health-related fitness and athletic proficiency can go together, but they are not synonymous to one another. Achieving health-related fitness is possible for (most) anyone who pursues it, regardless of one's ability to throw, catch, or kick a ball. Motor-skill proficiency can aid the development of health-related fitness, and motor skill practice is introduced here as a component that ought to be included in one's exercise routine but it is not required. This will be discussed later in more detail.

Third, you do not need to be a higher education student of kinesiology or exercise physiology or the like to understand the basic concepts of health-related fitness and what is required to achieve health-related benefit from physical activity participation. Clearly, the more knowledge the better, but once you comprehend the basic principles that underlie health-related achievement, you can ensure your compliance and foster the possible benefits.

Just What Is Health-Related Fitness?

Ancient civilizations advocated for physical activity participation, understanding the need for balance in one's life among what they considered the cognitive, spiritual, and physical. As if part of a three-legged stool, vigorous physical activity was considered one of the legs of wellness. Fast-forward several millennia, and the sentiment about physical activity's contribution to wellness continues to ring true; in fact, this sentiment is supported by more than lore or anecdotes, and we now understand from science its indisputable ability to contribute to our healthy well-being.

Simply, we now know that **physical activity participation can be health-protective!**

So, how? In what way?

Science has confirmed the amazing health-protective, health-related benefit that regular physical activity can yield:

- healthy blood pressure
- healthy blood sugar (reduced risk of diabetes)
- healthy body weight (reduced risk of overweight)
- healthy percentage of body fat (reduced risk of obesity)
- healthy bone density (reduced risk of osteoporosis)
- reduced risk of certain cancers
- healthy cholesterol (reduced risk of heart attack and stroke)
- healthy blood flow

In addition, engaging in physical activity also has the power to impact cognition and our emotional health. Certain markers include the following:

- enhanced cognitive function, e.g., attention
- enhanced self-esteem from maintaining a routine and realizing performance improvement
- release of endorphins which elicit the "runner's high"

- enhanced mood stability from releasing stress
- relief from anxiety and depression

Physical well-being is a product of cardiovascular and muscular proficiency, joint range-of-motion, and body composition (ratio of body fat tissue to lean muscle tissue). The health-related benefits that can be yielded from physical activity participation fall within the following categories and comprise the components of health-related fitness: cardiovascular health, muscular strength and muscular endurance, flexibility, and body composition.

All physical activity is not the same. Pursuing health-related fitness, engaging in physical activities such that health protection is stimulated, is typically different from pursuing performance-related fitness. It is also different from pursuing physical activity from a leisure perspective (meaning low intensity).

Possessing foot speed and a degree of agility and being able to throw a softball, for example, certainly can be indicators of possessing the ability to perform well in certain sports, *but neither taken alone offers health protection*. In order to reap the health-related benefit that physical activity participation can yield, we must abide by the principles that guide health-related fitness. That is, we must understand the ways in which we need to be physically active and be sure that each time we pass our key fob through the gym door or step outside for a run we *will* reap the benefit possible from that session of activity. This includes understanding the components that comprise health-related fitness and the protocol for achieving results related to each.

Considering the alternative, and the critically high stakes at hand (our well-being), how can any of us risk engaging in an exercise routine that in any way will compromise what can be gained? How can any of us take part in any activity or activity session in which health-related achievement is not the goal?

Health protection is enhanced when we engage in purposeful physical activities whereby the components of health-related fitness are addressed. Purposeful physical activities are those that actually[*] strengthen our heart, strengthen our muscles, help us to sustain joint flexibility, and help us to maintain a healthy ratio of body fat tissue to lean tissue. Thus help us to *achieve* in the realm of physical activity participation.

So What about the Physical Activity Routines We Develop?

Most of the gym-going population frames their exercise activity around the routines they have developed to structure their time once entering the facility or emerging from the locker room. Being creatures of habit, the routines we form quickly define our gym purpose and presence.

But our routine needs to be purposeful toward contributing to our physical well-being. This means doing what's required to strengthen your heart and muscles and impact your joint range-of-motion and body composition. Health-related fitness that yields health protection can be fostered through our physical activity participation *IF* we approach our engagement from an achievement perspective.

> **What an achievement perspective is:** an approach to your gym routine whereby you consistently engage according to what is required to yield the possible health-protective benefits of physical activity participation.

> **What an achievement perspective isn't:** thinking that gym achievement is only for those who possess elite athletic prowess; you don't need to be an accomplished competitive athlete to engage in physical activity that will yield health-protective benefits.

Basic Principles of Achievement-Oriented Health-Related Fitness

First, participating in any form of physical activity is better than being sedentary. Getting some activity is always better than getting no activity. But for optimal benefit we need to adhere to engagement that induces health protection. We owe it to our well-being to not settle for participation that is less than achievement-oriented.

Physical activity participation can be health-protective if its engagement is according to what's required to impact the components of health-related fitness (cardiovascular strength, muscular strength, muscular endurance, joint flexibility, and body composition). If its engagement is not according to what's required to induce impact, it might have been fun to do or a way to socialize with others, but it won't yield health protection. The leisurely stroll with the dog or visit to the park with your child may have great benefit, but it likely had little impact on the components of health-related fitness so vital to our well-being.

Second, health-related fitness is a topic that frames the sub-disciplines of college degree programs in kinesiology and related fields (physical education, wellness, nutritional science). As such, it carries its own knowledge base, the scope of such being too expansive to present here. The purpose of the following framework is to outline the basic principles that underlie achievement for each health-related fitness component. While what is presented is so in accordance to known science, the intent is to offer what is necessary for you to have a baseline understanding of the concepts.

Toward assessing the professional competency of your trainer, you can use this information to determine if the routine he/she prescribes in fact will yield health protection. Understanding what is required to induce health-related achievement is a critical piece of being an informed consumer. If there are big differences between what the principles outline and what your trainer prescribes then you are being trained to underachieve and it is time to hire a new trainer!

The following are the components of health-related fitness and their principles. Are these the principles your trainer is prescribing?

Cardiovascular Strength
Anchored by the heart muscle, our cardiovascular system pumps blood throughout our body and controls respiration. The healthier

our heart, the more efficient blood is pumped and in optimal volume. Similar to other muscles, the heart requires appropriate stimulation to sustain its strength. Engaging in aerobic physical activity elevates heart rate to provide the exertion necessary to yield health-protective benefit.

Many different types of activity can be aerobic and induce elevation including walking, running, cycling, spinning, participating in group aerobics (step, kick boxing, jazzercise, etc.), using cardio equipment (elliptical, stair master, stair mill), swimming, rowing, circuit training, skating (in-line or ice), and skiing (especially cross-country). The type of movement doesn't matter so long as a safely elevated heart rate is sustained for the recommended duration of time to foster cardiovascular benefit. Too much exertion and safety is compromised. Too little exertion and health benefit isn't stimulated. Appropriate heart rate is determined by the formula 220 – age (which indicates maximum heart rate), then 65-75 percent (heart rate training zone) of that number. For example, a fifty-year-old's maximum heart rate is 170 beats per minute (220–50), but the optimal heart rate training zone is between 110 and 127 beats per minute.

Current CDC recommendations call for accruing a minimum of 150 minutes of moderate or 75 minutes of vigorous, aerobic physical activity a week. Moderate activity is engagement at the lower end of the training zone, while vigorous activity is engagement at the higher end of the training zone. For greater cardiovascular benefit, 300 minutes of moderate or 150 minutes of vigorous activity ought to be completed a week.

These guidelines can help you gauge the amount of time you ought to engage in aerobic activity each day. They can also help you determine the professional capacity of your trainer or trainer-candidate. Is he/she aware of the guidelines? Does he/she ensure or advocate for obtaining the recommended duration of aerobic activity from you each week? And at the appropriate level of intensity?

Considering the benefit, *daily* cardiovascular activity ought to be prioritized.

Two methods for measuring your heart rate during exercise:

Purchase and use a heart rate monitor. Available at most well-stocked sporting goods store, some models offer basic functions while others include sophisticated features offering downloadable data, etc. Choose the model you are comfortable with then read the directions thoroughly so you assure the accuracy of the readout and understand the meaning of the readout numbers. Once you have completed any necessary data input, gaze at the readout as you engage in physical activity and adjust your intensity/effort as necessary.

OR

Use the time readout on the piece of cardio equipment you are using to count your heart rate. There are two options to monitor your heart-rate using this method:

1. *Count your heart rate for 10 seconds, then multiply that number by 6 to determine your beats per minute.* First, find your pulse either along your neck (ceratoid artery) or directly on your heart. (I find the heart location to have the stronger pulse, so I always use that one.) Begin your count with 1 when the time readout shows any number ending with 1 (1, 11, 21, 31, 41, 51, for example), then end your count when the readout reaches the subsequent number ending with 0. So if you begin your count at 1, end your count at 10; if you begin your count at 11, end your count at 20; if you begin your count at 21, end your count at 30, etc. Multiply that number by 6 to determine your heart rate according to the 1-minute standard.

2. *Count your heart rate for 6 seconds, then add a 0 to the end of that number to determine your beats per minute.* Begin your count when the time readout shows any number ending with 1 (see above), then end your count when the readout

reaches the subsequent number ending with 6. So if you begin your count at 1, end your count at 6; if you begin your count at 11, end your count at 16; if you begin your count at 21, end your count at 26, etc. Then, add a zero to the end of the number to determine your heart rate according to the 1-minute standard.

Note: most pieces of cardio equipment come equipped with a heart rate feature. Users hold onto sensors for a certain period of time until the determined heart rate is displayed. While the readout may be accurate, I suggest using either of the methods described above to ensure accuracy. Appropriate exertion is critical toward reaping the intended cardiovascular benefit. Don't rely on what MIGHT be accurate.

Points to Consider

- In the name of cardio, exercisers often are instructed by trainers to go for a certain distance or a certain amount of time. Simply covering a certain distance or engaging for a certain amount of time does not mean that optimal cardiovascular gains will be fostered—unless it is accomplished while in the heart rate training zone. Otherwise, walking on the treadmill means just that—walking on the treadmill.

- Second, the so-called warm-up, or time it takes to get your heart rate into its training zone, should not count toward the minimum amount of time needed each session to promote cardiovascular benefit, especially when intending vigorous engagement. To ensure that you reap cardiovascular benefit, begin to note your accumulation of time *after* your heart rate has entered its training zone (of moderate or vigorous intensity).

- Last, cardiovascular disease (coronary heart disease, stroke, hypertension, and congestive heart failure) is a leading cause of death in the United States, and the related medical cost was estimated to be $297.7 billion in

2008.[2]* Regular physical activity, engaged in according to one's training zone, can prevent cardiovascular disease.

Muscular Strength and Muscular Endurance

The muscular system serves to enable movement. In concert with the central nervous system, skeletal muscles pull against bones to produce movement. Muscles also enable posture and protect vital organs. The more muscular strength and endurance we possess, the easier it is to go about the physical tasks that comprise our lives. Albeit less so than previous generations given advances in mechanism and technology, the physicality of daily life can be extensive: getting in and out of the car, getting in and out of chairs, shuttling kids to school, grocery shopping, doing the wash, cleaning the house, etc. These common tasks require some degree of muscular strength and/or endurance to accomplish. Developed muscular qualities can profoundly impact quality of life for how they impact the ability to simply move through the day.

Beyond consideration for how we move about the day, muscular strength and endurance can impact the physical activity in which we participate outside the gym. The quality with which we can engage in any activity is enhanced upon developing greater strength and endurance. Muscular qualities also impact our body composition (ratio of lean body tissue to fat) in that lean mass can be increased and fat decreased through appropriate training. The greater the ratio of lean mass to fat, the healthier our composition.

Improving muscular strength or endurance requires resistance training (weight training) during which weights are used to *overload* muscles (make muscles or muscle groups put forth more energy than usual). Resistance training is conducted by completing a certain number of repetitions of an exercise for a certain number of times (sets) for each muscle or muscle group targeted. In general, completing 5–7 repetitions of an exercise promotes *strength* gains, while completing 10–12 repetitions promotes *endurance* gains. The resistance has to overload the muscle which means using a HEAVY enough weight so that the last repetition of a set is barely possible. This is appropriate overload that will stimulate muscular gains! Muscles are remarkable for their ability to adapt to stresses, meaning muscles will strengthen by training them to strengthen. Muscles need progressive stress (heavier and heavier) to stimulate further gains in strength and endurance.

The CDC recommends a minimum of two strength-training days a week, with each major muscle group being targeted for one set of 8–12 repetitions. The major muscles to target include pecs, deltoids, lats, biceps/triceps, quads, glutes, and hamstrings. At least forty-eight hours should separate strength-training sessions of any muscle to allow sufficient time for the muscle to regenerate. For example, if pecs are targeted on Monday, they shouldn't be targeted again until at least Wednesday.

Additional muscular benefit can be realized by increasing the number of strength-training sessions per week or number of sets completed for each muscle. Quality trainers be able to establish a strength-training routine that appropriately takes rest time into consideration (the time between sessions that target specific muscles) as well as the protocol to stimulate strength and endurance. Back-to-back days working a specific muscle or muscle group are counter to fostering muscular gains and can even lead to injury. This also means that group exercise classes that include a strength-training circuit have to be factored into the strength-training scheme. Whether done as part of a group class that also promotes cardiovascular work or as a stand-alone session, targeting the same muscle or muscle group two days in a row should be avoided.

Note to women: due to hormonal differences (comparably less testosterone), women are not able to gain muscle mass like men do (unless chemically augmented). But when women follow the appropriate training protocol, they will develop a degree of muscle mass—and this is a GOOD THING!

Considering how mass adds a degree of protection to our skel-etal structure, related both to protecting our organs and bone density, mass is extremely important to our vitality. Bone is organic matter that has to be stimulated to generate (or maintain) density. The greater the density, the less likely that breaks will occur. Stimulation to induce density is generated by muscles pulling against bones as it occurs during physical activity. Weight-bearing exercise (i.e., walking, running, forms of group aerobic classes) and resistance training requires muscles to pull against bones for movement to be executed. These types of activ-ity can especially contribute to the bone health of our hips and spine. But whether through weight-bearing exercise or resistance training, the greater the mass of the muscle pulling against the bone, the more the bone can develop girth as a response.[3*]

Resistance training to foster strength, endurance, AND mass can counteract the impact aging has on bone density. According to the National Osteoporosis Foundation, 25 million people in the United States are afflicted with osteoporosis, including one-half of all women over the age of fifty. The research is indisputable—bone density can at least be maintained by consistently including resistance training as part of a regimen that also addresses nutrition and vitamin and mineral supplementation. Muscle mass, ladies, is a good thing! We ought to do as much as possible to develop and maintain as much bone density as possible.

Most of us would rather look robust than not, because along with the look comes a degree of healthfulness. And much more im-portant than the look of our physique is how what we have done to achieve our physique has contributed to our health! Robust, appealing physiques are achieved by engaging in physical activity appropriate to what is required to maximize heart health, and musculature, and mini-mize body fat. Being robust is a good thing, and muscle mass contrib-utes to robustness.

Health-related achievement related to muscular quality does not include 'shaping', 'toning', and/or contour-ing. Each implies a goal that grossly neglects the health impacting development of strength, endurance and mass. Each also represents the pursuit of ambiguous outcomes—that likely are never realized—and so dangerously undermine motivation. Due to hormonal make up women respond differently than men to resistance training, but the purpose for doing so is gender neutral.

Flexibility

The manner in which we move is greatly influenced by the range of motion of our joints and the suppleness of our soft tissue (including muscles). Be it our knees, elbows, hips, neck, or ankles, joints that have limited range of motion and muscles that have reduced elasticity will profoundly compromise the quality of our movement. Flexibility is the degree to which our joints and soft tissue maintain optimal range of motion.

Efficient physical movement is rhythmic and flowing. Having compromised range of motion or otherwise being "inflexible" or "tight" can contribute to movement that is herky-jerky, lopsided, unbalanced, and painful. Joint range of motion can be compromised by neglecting to engage in flexibility exercises, by degenerative diseases such as arthritis, and/or by damage such as cartilage tears. If afflicted by disease or damage, a flexibility routine may not restore range of motion but it can aid the maintenance of range of motion as best possible.

Flexibility can be best maintained by engaging in both static (not moving) and dynamic (moving) stretching. These types of movements are also important to prepare our bodies for progressively intense physical activity and to prevent injury. Any bout of activity ought to be preceded by a warm-up, some light activity to promote blood flow, to get the blood moving throughout the body. The warm-up ought to include 2–3 minutes of moderate aerobic activity (a light jog, moderate walk on the treadmill, moderate time on the elliptical, etc.) followed by dynamic stretching. A dynamic stretching routine can consist of leg pendulum swings (to the front and side), high-knee walking/marching, glute kicks, and big arm circles. Dynamic stretching does not include holding poses for a certain amount of time. This is static stretching, which ought to be done to *conclude* a physical activity session. Static stretching includes holding poses whereby all major muscles are stretched to induce lengthening. Working from top to bottom, at minimum, static stretches should "hit" the shoulders/pecs, triceps, quads, hamstrings, glutes, and calves.

Points to Consider

- Mind-body exercising (i.e., yoga, pilates, etc.) has become popular in recent years. While these are powerful forms of physical activity, forsaking other forms of activity and only doing these types of exercises <u>will</u> compromise your overall health-related achievement. In general, this type of activity especially will not yield the same cardiovascular benefit as aerobic activity.

- At the other end of the spectrum, don't neglect to consistently include stretching as part of a health-related fitness routine. At stake is preserving structural alignment and the suppleness of soft tissue, which diminishes through aging. Without regular stretching it is more likely that range of motion will be diminished more and much earlier than if we consistently address this aspect of our physical well-being. Further, without regularly stretching we are at much greater risk for injury and thus needing to take time off from activity. The physical health ramifications of having to take time off speak for themselves, but perhaps under-considered yet equally as impactful is the emotional toll that time away can induce. The stress relief that physical activity participation can provide ought never be taken for granted or undervalued. Every day brings with it stress that needs to be burned off in as healthful a manner as possible.

- Last, there is the potential for one-time injuries or annoying conditions to turn into nagging or chronic issues that require professional care if an appropriate flexibility routine is not followed. For example, 70–80 percent of adults experience low back pain at some point in their lives[4*]. Exercises that target the abdominals and back muscles and stretching are typically included to both treat and prevent low back pain. Considering how pervasive this condition is within the adult population, it alone makes the case for consistently addressing flexibility as part of one's health-related fitness routine.

Body Composition

Body weight may or may not indicate healthfulness because its measure includes both lean mass tissue (muscle, bones, organs) and fat. For health protection, the greater the ratio of lean mass to fat mass, the generally healthier one is. Achieving healthy body composition requires exerting enough energy throughout the day to burn the food calories we ingest <u>and</u> engaging in physical activity such that we build our lean mass.

Besides the protective benefit to our heart, aerobic exercise is also critical to our health-related fitness for its ability to burn calories. If we burn the calories that we ingest, we can maintain our body weight and control or over time reduce our body fat. Excessive calories are stored as fat. The result of not burning the calories that we ingest is an increase in body weight and increase in body fat. Excessive body weight can unduly stress soft tissue while excessive body fat increases the risk for obesity-related disease. Maintaining body weight is typically a point of energy balance—calories in mitigated by calories burned (stated with due reverence to those challenged by the presence of disease or related condition whereby body weight cannot be regulated by energy balance).

Building lean mass requires engaging in physical activity that will foster muscular development—growth. As presented previously, resistance or weight training is what will appropriately overload our muscles to stimulate growth. It can also yield health protection by contributing to healthy body composition, making the importance of achieving muscular development all the more important.

Points to Consider

- Looks can be deceiving when it comes to determining how the physical appearance of someone or their body weight may or may not accurately indicate their level of healthfulness for the primary reason that lean mass weighs more than fat mass (muscle weighs more than fat). For example, picture two women who both stand at 5'4" and to the naked eye appear to have similar physiques and wear the same size. One woman, though, weighs 120 pounds and carries 20 percent body fat, while the other woman weighs 130 pounds and carries 12 percent body fat. All things equal, the one weighing more has more lean tissue than the other and so has a comparatively healthier body composition.

- There is much more to the numbers of weight than meets the eye. What makes up the numbers is what matters to health protection. Accurately determining a valid measure of healthfulness based upon body weight alone is not possible unless further assessment to determine body composition also is included. Further, even if one's body weight is in the so-called healthy zone (insurance companies still use weight-relative-to-height charts to determine one aspect of our health), the composition of the weight may in fact render a person terribly unhealthy. Or vice-versa.

  BMI, or Body Mass Index is a calculation based upon a ratio between height and weight that estimates body fat. BMI calculators can be easily accessed on the internet.

- With some latitude given, the following illustrates the qualitative differences between lean tissue and fatty tissue. Excessive fat is like the bullying weed in the garden—it has no redeemable social graces or sense of boundaries and annoyingly springs up wherever it can. Excessive fat is only a taker, but certain strategies can be employed to keep its growth at bay. Fat cells are proverbial web-surfing, video-playing, sedentary couch potatoes. While muscles get up and get going, fat only observes life as it occurs around its orb. While its gnarled root system will not ever entirely disappear, it can be kept hidden underground through consistent effort (regular health-related physical activity) so as not to subject others to its ugliness. Muscle is like the warm sun—it nourishes, stimulates growth, and promotes well-being for what it has the capacity to do: produce movement. Muscle is a giver. Unlike fat cells that are comparatively dormant, muscle cells are active and organic. Muscle cells participate in life because they live themselves.

- Last,_building muscle mass can contribute to a metabolism boost (burning more energy, thus aiding healthy body composition), but the boost is relatively small because in most cases the mass that is built is not large enough to enact a significant change. Enhanced muscular strength ought to be prioritized because *stronger* muscles especially impact metabolism.

Summary

We owe it to ourselves to ensure that we engage in physical activity that is *health-related* and *achievement-oriented*. Health-related fitness routines need exercises that will strengthen the heart, strengthen and build muscles, improve joint range of motion, and decrease body fat.

We also owe it to ourselves to make sure that the gym routine we establish or that is established for us by a personal trainer appropriately and adequately addresses each health-related component. Otherwise, under-activity, ineffective activity (related to health protection), and underachieving activity can cost our pocketbook and most importantly our quality of life.

The section above provides one source of information useful toward assessing the *competency* of your fitness professional. What follows is a second source of information specific to ascertaining an indication of the trainer's *attitude* and *aptitude* toward conducting personal training. Armed with a baseline understanding of health-related fitness content knowledge, combined with the described protocol to hire a trainer or determine if you will continue with your current trainer you will confidently be able to ensure the quality of your fitness professional and be an informed consumer.

II. Assessing the Professional Competency of Your Trainer or Trainer-Candidate

These are points to consider and keep in mind as you assess and reassess the fitness professional with whom you are working, particularly regarding your *achievement* at the gym. If your trainer exhibits any of the following or your intuition leads you to believe he/she is deficient in any of the concepts examined that is a red flag you need to respond to immediately and without hesitation.

When you join a gym, the gym may offer an option to purchase a personal training package delivered by one of that gym's training cadre. And of course at any time thereafter you can always buy into a package. By all means, if you feel that a trainer would enhance your relationship with physical activity and thus make it more likely that you would reap the possible health-related benefits, then don't delay even for a moment. Hire a trainer and hit the ground running!

But hiring a *competent* trainer is easier said than done. Most gym facilities tend to do little to facilitate the process other than to "match" you to one who is available. Many gyms have a picture board of their trainers with a description of their credentials and training philosophies. True, from this you could get a sense of their professional preparation and a general feel for their style and/or focus. But beyond the paragraph that describes their training outlook, it's impossible to garner further information. Your health-related wellness deserves a selection process that entails a little more than chance, one that will match you with a training professional who can competently guide your achievement. Again, considering the stakes, buyer beware is certainly relevant!

So, how can you go about making this important decision?

The following two-part process is a systematic means to assess a trainer-candidate's content knowledge, philosophy, and professional demeanor (aptitude and attitude). The interview is intended to help you understand the candidate's personal and professional background with physical activities and training and how that plays out in his/her delivery. Theory and reality sometimes being incongruent, though, the trial training session is intended to understand the reality of the candidate's approach. We all know that communicating our beliefs and philosophies can be one thing, but what occurs in application can be another. I hate to say it, but in the interest of attaining clients, I have overheard trainers telling prospects seemingly what they think the clients want to hear. The selection process ought to ferret out inconsistencies that hopefully will lead to you hiring the best candidate.

The suggested questions and subsequent responses are provided specifically mindful of the *achievement-oriented health-related fitness* approach that underlies this book. Remember, you don't need someone just to act as your gym host guiding you through the motions and chatting with you. You need someone who will help you reap the health-protective benefits that are possible through physical activity participation. You need someone who understands what it takes to achieve health-related fitness and who can solicit achievement responses.

Even though you may be new to the realm of achievement-oriented physical activity and feel you don't have adequate preparation yourself to assess a trainer-candidate, my guess is that you have had plenty of related experience to successfully negotiate this process. You likely have had to engage in processes both at work and at home to assess the professional capacity of others—co-workers, clients, baby sitters, teachers, etc. For any of these scenarios you likely systematically gathered the relevant information possible and then acted accordingly. The same scrutiny is necessary here—after all, he/she is going to become YOUR co-worker, client, and care-giver of sorts.

And perhaps as in the other similar scenarios, your instincts kicked in once the process started. Listen closely to the responses from the trainer-candidate, observe his/her demeanor in responding and delivering a session, but also pay attention to what your gut is telling you. You don't have to be an expert in exercise physiology to realize that someone is inconsistent, unpleasant, or inattentive. These are blatant red flags indicative of professional conduct that will not go away.

One last thing about the trainer-client relationship before moving on to the process. Keep in mind that you are the client and, as such, you control whether your trainer remains in your employ (considering the contract you establish, of course). Not the gym, not the trainer, not your friends, you. *You* decide if your trainer is in fact aiding your progress or not. If not, do not waste any time before pursuing someone else. The great news is that there are fabulous trainers ready to help you achieve.

Two-Step Process to Help Determine the Professional Capacity of a Trainer:

1. Interview the trainer-candidate to garner responses to the questions below. This will help you acquire information about his/her philosophy, experience, and communication skills. If the trainer-candidate is reluctant to take the time to interview or seems bothered by the inconvenience, well, the boldest of red flags would have already reared its true color.

    During the interview listen carefully to the responses, especially for specifics and examples, and pay attention to the body language—comfortable? annoyed? engaging? What is displayed relays pertinent information about the candidate that you should carefully scrutinize.

2. Engage in a trial training session delivered by your trainer-candidate (for a reduced cost). This will help you gauge his/her professional demeanor and determine the trainer's degree of consistency between what he/she espouses (gathered from the interview) to what he/she actually de-

livers. To this, physical activity professionals tend to be very consistent in their delivery of instruction/leadership from one session to the next. Therefore, doing a trial of even one session ought to provide valuable insight to help establish if he/she possesses the competency necessary to deliver results. The trial session ought to match the same time duration as a "real" session to enable you to garner as much "real" information as possible.

Step One: Interview Your Trainer-Candidate
What to Ask and What Responses to Look for and Watch Out for

Why are you a trainer? How did you get into training?

What to look for:

- *"Sense of Mission"*
  In other words, a love of and for physical activity, including his or her own life history of participation in varied types of physical activity. Also, reference to being drawn to training others after he/she himself/herself had a profound health-related experience, i.e., losing significant weight or going through a health scare that induced them to make lifestyle changes.

- *"Additional source of income"*
  Reality being what it is, many of us seek opportunities to earn extra income. Moonlighting as a trainer can be a terrific source of income. This would be especially prudent if the candidate was already employed in the physical activity enterprise (e.g., physical education teacher, recreation leader).

- *"I like working with people and helping them attain health-related outcomes."*
  This response is related to regarding this work as one's mission. Effective trainers ought to be as committed to your health-related fitness as you are. One caveat to this

point, though. It goes without saying, but inherent to the training process is a high degree of interaction between trainer and client. While an interest in "working with people" is an obvious motivator toward entering this work, the professional preparation has to match the interest. Don't fall prey to one who is well intended (great from an interactive perspective) but who is unprepared to deliver achievement-oriented health-related fitness outcomes.

What to watch out for:

- *Any reference to or indication of not knowing what other profession to pursue*
  Essentially holding onto the "glory days" of playing high school/college sports and seemingly not being able to move beyond—professionally speaking. The troublesome dynamic is one who might feel this is their only viable professional option. Instead of entering the field, driven by a sense of passion or mission, it is by default. The resulting emotional connection of regret or resentment may always cloud the commitment one can make to the profession and clientele.

- *Any indication of personality traits of possession, control, or pent-up resentment toward punitive physical activity leaders from their past*
  Your achievement-oriented health-related fitness journey needs to be about you. A trainer ought to indicate his/her sense of ownership toward your goals, but not to the extent that his/her goals become your goals or that a "my way or the highway" atmosphere will be created. Your health-related fitness is *your* health-related fitness. Similarly, you ought to avoid a trainer who seems to indicate he/she relishes telling people what to do for the sake of telling people what to do.

What are your qualifications?

What to look for:

- *A degree in physical education, kinesiology, health, wellness, or related field is preferred along with a fitness certification (personal trainer certification) from a reputable[5*] source*
  In the realm of physical activity leadership, content knowledge is *the* primary tangible that separates an "expert" leader from an "effective" one. The more content knowledge a trainer accrues, the more likely it is he/she possesses a comprehensive understanding of the training process and an extensive repertoire of exercises and workout plans. This also makes it more likely he/she will offer prudent feedback and provide accurate assessments. College degree programs typically require at least two years of coursework specific to a major.

  In addition to a degree, a fitness certification from a reputable[*] source provides content knowledge focused upon the art and science of personal training. But, as was mentioned earlier, certification programs differ greatly in what is required to be deemed "certified" as a personal trainer. Some can be completed over a weekend, some are completed online, and others are longer-term and require both cognitive and practical components. Keeping in mind that content knowledge is *the* factor separating the best from the okay, it would be prudent to ascertain your potential trainer's perspective on his/her preparation.

- *Indication of an interest in working with people to help them attain health-related outcomes*
  This is a given, a "has to," an imperative part of the training relationship about to be forged. As stated, the trainer-candidate ought to be as interested in your outcomes as you are, and this interest ought to clearly emerge during the course of your conversation. There is no substitute for possessing and operating from this perspective. If you at all detect this to be deficient, or question the trainer-candidate's intent, move along to the next candidate. This simply can not be otherwise compensated for, so don't make any excuse for the deficiency.

What to watch out for:

- *Dismissing the question about his/her qualifications*
  One's own history of physical activity participation certainly can enhance one's capacity to be an effective trainer.
  After all, understanding what the trainee is experiencing
  can prompt the trainer to utilize motivational techniques
  appropriately aligned to the trainee's level of performance.
  But professional preparation includes more than knowing
  one's way around a gym based upon one's own experience
  in said gym. Also, just because one can "do," doesn't mean
  that one can inspire another to do. Among other dynam-
  ics, a trainer-candidate with limited preparation other than
  his/her own training likely will instruct the trainee to follow
  his/her routine or protocol. It might be that the protocol
  would in fact foster health-related fitness outcomes, but
  chances are otherwise. For one, the trainer-candidate's
  protocol may be deficient in certain health-related fitness
  components, without the trainer even knowing or caring.
  Secondly, given genetics, each of us has a unique response
  to training. True, the principles of health-related fitness
  are universal, but we may have a natural propensity for
  flexibility more so than muscular strength, etc. Sharing a
  similar genetic make-up as the trainer-candidate is highly
  unlikely. Therefore, abiding by his/her routine likely would
  not serve you well. Without adequate, quality professional
  preparation, trainers can come to conduct their training
  practice according to how they were trained—the teach-
  how-you-have-been-taught phenomenon. If lucky, one's
  trainer will have experienced quality training themselves,
  and thus operate accordingly to the benefit of the trainees.
  Most likely, though, the training protocol one's trainer experienced was deficient.

The primary point here is to not leave one's own training
process to chance.
There may be no substitute for experience, but there defi-
nitely is no substitute for professional preparation. If your
trainer-candidate in any way dismisses the necessity of for-

mal preparation this is a blatant red flag indicating deficient professional capacity.

Please describe your philosophy about personal training/attaining fitness.

What to look for:

- *Decisive acknowledgment that each of the components of health-related fitness are addressed during sessions or over the course of a series of sessions*

- *Indication that health-related markers/goals underlie the purpose of the training process (not goals based on appearance)*

- *Indication that sessions are planned, thus purposeful*

- *Indication of an approach that is guided by the scientific principles known to induce health-related benefit*

- *Indication that physical activity participation ought to be a daily habit—so encouragement to reap the quality-of-life benefit of physical activity participation daily*

- *Indication that regular assessment is conducted to ascertain information about achievement*

- *Indication of being an aid/partner toward your efforts to own your health-related fitness process*

- *The mention of a training process that is specific to your age and present level of fitness/activity*

- *The mention of protocol used to ensure the safety of the training process, including an initial assessment to determine your present level of fitness*

What to watch out for:

- *Making promises for/guaranteeing radical body transformation or indicating that the process can result in body parts looking like a celebrity's—i.e., "arms like Angelina Jolie's"*

- *Suggesting that the process will be easy*

- *Suggesting a "magic pill" approach or that by doing "one specific thing" goals will be met and discounting the need for a balanced approach to training—i.e., just one kind of circuit work or weight work*

- *Differentiating between men's and women's fitness goals—i.e., men lift heavy weights to get strong, women lift light weights to tone*

- *Diminishing/discounting the training process for older individuals*

- *Providing advice about diet/nutrition—unless possessing reputable credentials, such as proof of college-level nutritional science coursework*

- *Disparaging the manner in which other trainers conduct their sessions or the philosophies they hold*

- *Presuming an understanding of your goals, especially based upon gender—i.e., women wanting to work on "trouble spots"*

Have you/do you train women/men (depending upon your [the trainee's] gender)?

What to look for:

- *"Yes."   Which can then prompt further follow-up questions from you (see below)*

- *"No."*   *Which can indicate a simple lack of opportunity to do so prior to now or a professional outlook that indicates a disturbing professional perspective (see below)*
  If the response is due to lack of previous opportunity then his/her subsequent responses to the questions that follow will provide additional insight into his/her capacity to be a good match for you.

What to watch out for:

- *Demeaning the attitude or aptitude a gender projects towards training—i.e., "women don't know what they are doing," "men are too aggressive."*
  While it certainly is any trainer's prerogative as to the clientele they establish, discounting an entire gender with a generalized perception reflects narrow perspective, lack of experience, and rigidness.

If you train both genders what differences, if any, do you employ while training either?

What to look for:

- *Indication that the training protocol delivered is the same for both genders*

- *Indication that the scientific principles that underlie health-related fitness are gender-neutral*

- *Indication of the expectation of achievement whether training men or women*

What to watch out for:

- *Overt or covert reference to attitude or aptitude differences between men and women that perpetuate stereotypical myths, i.e, men will not stretch (so I won't have them work on joint range of motion), women do not want to bulk up (so I won't* have them lift heavy weights), or any indication of presumed fitness goals or approach to training based upon gender, i.e., women steered toward cardio, men steered toward weights

- Using different descriptors for women than men to outline training objectives, i.e., training women to "tone" while training men to "bulk up"

- Indicating a focus upon "fixing" so-called "trouble spots" for women, including the reference that spot-reduction is possible, i.e., losing weight in hips or buttocks exclusively

Have you/do you train clients my age?

What to look for:

- "Yes."   Follow up this response by asking the two related questions below.

- "No."   This response can indicate a simple lack of opportunity to do so prior to now, or that the trainer-candidate is not interested in working with clients your age.
Likely this would not be the case given he/she is talking to you about being your trainer, but obviously if this is the case then proceed to the next candidate. If the response is due to lack of previous opportunity then his/her subsequent responses to the questions that follow below will provide additional insight into his/her capacity to be a good match for you.

What to watch out for:

- Demeaning the interest in training of a specific population— i.e., seniors by using dumbed-down language or otherwise projecting the attitude that seniors are not serious trainees

- Dismissing the question by projecting a one-size-fits-all approach to training

While the principles that underlie health-related fitness achievement can be generalized across the life span, science has informed discernment for how the principles are to be modified according to age. One size does not fit all when considering training protocol across the life span. One's safety could be sorely at risk if a trainer is not aware of the parameters of training for individuals of different ages. Content knowledge is especially pertinent for how it informs training protocol across the life span.

What do you know to be the main health issues facing someone my age and how can physical activity participation impact these issues?

What to look for:

- *Response(s) that include reference to bone health, hormonal changes (and how it impacts mood, bone health, heart health), loss of muscle strength/mass, compromised balance, joint health, propensity to gain weight/body fat due to metabolic changes, and loss of independence due to diminished physical capability*

- *Responses to the second part of the question that clearly describe how physical activity can help to mitigate certain health issues*
  For example, weight-bearing exercise and bone health (hopefully also reference to muscles needing to pull against bone to stimulate growth), resistance training and muscle mass maintenance, exercise and mood stability, exercise and balance maintenance, exercise and metabolism, exercise and the preservation of lean muscle mass, stretching and the preservation of joint range-of-motion, and exercise and daily independence—e.g., carrying groceries, mobility, caring for one's home.

What to watch out for:

- *Inability to identify the main health issues facing men or women of certain ages*

A lack of awareness of the key health issues that are pertinent to specific populations of men and women indicates insufficient content knowledge. This can be the result of inadequate professional preparation or ongoing professional development.

- *Indication that physical activity participation can deliver a fountain of youth*
  While regular, health-related physical activity participation IS health protective and CAN aid to stave the physical capability diminishment that age can trigger, aging happens whether we like it or not and along with it some realities that impact our physical selves. Sixty-year-old knees tend to not function like twenty-year-old knees no matter our dedication to our health-related routine. Purporting the benefit of physical activity participation across one's lifetime—yes! Denying aging's impact on our participation—no!

Note: The preceding questions (*Have you/do you train men/ women?*, *Have you/do you train clients my age?*, and *What do you know to be the main health issues facing someone my age and how can physical activity participation impact these issues?*) are also helpful in ascertaining if the trainer-candidate possesses both content knowledge and experience to ask the right questions, as well as accurately respond to the questions clients pose.

Knowing what questions to ask of a specific population or age group can solicit critical information relative to fostering health-related fitness. Akin to seeing a healthcare specialist rather than a generalist, the specialist is going to be all the more familiar with nuances, motivational stances, and useful communication style.

Further, given the option, most of us will choose the professional who has conducted a necessary procedure multiple times rather than just a few times—we want the doctor who has repeatedly done a procedure or treated a condition. We go to seafood restaurants not burger joints for fish and seek hairstylists who are especially adept at styling the type of hair we possess—long, short, curly, thin, thick, etc.

So follows the thought of utilizing a fitness professional who possesses content knowledge and experience working with clientele similar to you. Knowing what questions to ask you can be equally important as accurately responding to those you pose. This implies that the trainer-candidate possesses content knowledge and experience and has engaged in professional reflection to ascertain for him/herself what works, what doesn't, and what needs to be adjusted in the course of fostering the health-related fitness of a certain sub-set of clientele.

What do you consider to be your significant accomplishment(s) as a trainer?

What to look for:

- *Decisively noting the specific health-related improvements that past or present clients have experienced*
  For example, improved aspects of heart health such as blood pressure, muscular strength gains, and body composition improvement. Also, noting the motor skill development of clients.

- *A response that takes the tone of "I am here to help my clients foster health-related gains, and/or gym achievement"*

- *A response that indicates improvement to past or present clients' relationship to physical activity or motivation to be physically active*
  Physical activity participation is driven by the motivation to be physically active. Motivation is commonly predicated by success. If a trainer is able to impact motivation, it follows that the trainer has been able to aid a client's achievement. This indicates a trainer who possesses the professional capacity to foster results.

What to watch out for:

- *An account of WHOM they have trained (ie., a certain celebrity, athlete, etc.), rather than what health-related gains they have helped foster in others*
  Especially in certain geographical areas of the country, trainers may seek to gain notoriety by becoming part of the inner circle of celebrities/public figures. Notoriety, though, ought to be the result of fostering achievement-oriented fitness results rather than simply becoming aligned to a public figure. A trainer-candidate ought to be as committed to your health-related fitness as you are, regardless of your public status or presenting level of fitness.

- *A response that is slow to formulate or defensive*
  A trainer-candidate ought to understand that the value of his/her professional merit is foremost determined by clients' health-related gains. This means clearly and without hesitation articulating the health-related gains that clients have made.

  If the trainer-candidate is annoyed with the question or takes on an "I don't have to prove anything to you" stance, this is indication of their professional immaturity.

- *A response that speaks more to relationships built with clients than how clients have realized health-related gains*
  Trainers need to possess strong interpersonal skills considering the time spent with clients—both frequency and duration—and potential for intimate relationships to develop (not suggesting sexualized), but not at the expense of eliciting health-related fitness gains. Be leery of a trainer-candidate who speaks about their clientele/work from a relationship focus. We don't need a gym host/hostess to keep us company; we need a proficiently prepared fitness professional to guide our health-related achievement. Consider the relationship you have with your doctors. Of course we prefer ones who possess pleasant "bedside manner," but more so we seek those whose preparation

and experience has yielded their aptitude to accurately help us sustain our health. The consideration for a trainer is the same.

Is your schedule amenable to taking on a new client?

What to look for:

- *Decisively and clearly indicating YES, followed by framing the days/times of availability*

What to watch out for:

- *Hemming and hawing about being able to juggle current commitments to "fit you in"*

On the one hand, being busy is some indication of quality. After all, the training environment (gym) tends to be a public domain and along with it a trainer's reputation. Even with limited knowledge about what constitutes "good" training, most of us will not tolerate someone we think is poor. On the other hand, though, your health-related well-being has to be as important to your trainer as it is with his/her other clients. Especially over time, being able to "fit you in" likely just isn't going to create the degree of attention necessary to fully commit to eliciting your health-related achievement.

Also, if the trainer-candidate is trying to "fit you in," he/she may water down the length of time of sessions or in one way or another allude to the fact that short sessions (i.e., twenty minutes rather than sixty minutes because his/her schedule will only permit this) are adequate. To be sure, some health-related fitness gains can be realized in shorter sessions and some physical activity is always better than no physical activity, but the degree of gains realized, and thus health protection, is underlain by the frequency of sessions and duration of each session. Twenty-minute sessions can be useful toward inducing cardiovascular benefit, but if you are also trying to induce muscular strength or joint range of motion gains twenty minutes likely is not adequate time to sufficiently address these multiple goals. Certain exceptions may exist, but in general and especially considering that most sessions with trainers are focused upon more than one health-related component, over time shorter sessions will yield less health-related gain as compared to longer sessions.

Further, a trainer-candidate who proposes shorter sessions likely also approaches training from a "just" perspective—as in you *just* need to do some cardio, or some weights, or some stretching, etc. A "just" perspective sorely discounts the scientific principles that underlie health-related fitness achievement. It also purports a haphazard, purposeless approach to sessions. In this case, failing to abide by the principles that guide fitness achievement will significantly diminish the benefits gained. The result? You just won't fully achieve the benefits possible.

Last, given established clientele who have dedicated sessions, the trainer-candidate may propose one long session a week (i.e., ninety minutes rather than fifty minutes) rather than multiple sessions spread out over the course of the week. Consistency is a key tenet of health-related fitness, meaning we need to consider the health-related physical activity we accrue on a DAILY basis. You may be able to guide your own activity for the days you are not working with your trainer, and this may be your ultimate goal from the outset, but if your physical activity participation only will occur when you are able to work with your trainer, once a week is not adequate frequency to induce optimal benefit (health protection).

What do you expect from your clients? What can I expect from you?

What to look for:

*   *Decisively and concisely describing the policies, procedures, and protocol of the training process*
    This ought to include specifics about what a typical session entails and policies about cancelled sessions or sessions

when you arrive late. This also ought to include reference to "you give me your best and I will give you my best."

- *Indication of shared power and intent to teach you how to sustain health-related fitness*
Bottom line, your health-related fitness is YOUR health-related fitness. Trainers serve an important role in the process but ought to work toward empowering the clients they serve to be able to foster their own gains. After all, trainers may come and go. To best serve your long-term interest, a trainer-candidate ought to have the intent and capacity to teach you how to reap the potential benefits.

What to watch out for:

- *Confusion about why you would pose the questions or dismissing the questions altogether*
This indicates a trainer-candidate who hasn't considered the questions, delivers sessions that are haphazardly planned, or doesn't care what you bring to the process. All point to a disregard for you, the client, a clear lack of professionalism, and deficient content knowledge. If you are an under-conditioned gym beginner, an ego-driven trainer who possesses comprehensive content knowledge could prove effective as you begin your fitness-related journey. But as time marches on the effectiveness will wane unless your perspective about the process and/or desired outcomes becomes more about you and less about he/she. The training process ought to NEVER be arbitrary—that is "sometimes this and sometimes that" during your sessions. Thanks to an extensive research community we understand the health-protective benefits of physical activity participation and the protocol for reaping them. A quality trainer is able to both explain how protocol plays itself out in the sessions they conduct and ensure that each session is conducted in accordance to the principles known to foster benefit.

What results can I expect from the training process?

(Note—The response to this question can be particularly significant for how it impacts your motivation. If (unrealistic) intended results are not realized then your motivation to adhere to your routine will wane. Eventually, sadly sooner than later, the disappointment caused by not realizing the identified results will erode your interest to continue to engage.)

What to look for:

- *Reference to health-related fitness gains (improvement)*
  It is essential to our well-being that we engage in physical activity such that our cardiovascular, muscular and skeletal systems benefit. An achievement-oriented, health-related fitness approach to physical activity will pave the way for improved cardiovascular strength, muscular strength and endurance, flexibility, and body composition. Well prepared, competent trainers understand this ought to be the focus that drives the training process, and the frame upon which results are pursued. A reference to body transformation is realistic to expect from the trainer-candidate, but only after health-related gains are mentioned. Health-related fitness improvement ought to underscore the trainer-candidate's intent and approach to your results.

  Related, the trainer-candidate also ought to mention the benefits that can be yielded upon (most) any physical activity engagement, e.g., stress relief, endorphin release, improved mood, and improved cognitive function.

- *A conservative time frame in which to expect body transformation*
  Body transformation (appearance change) can occur but over time, never overnight. Professionally-competent trainers understand that transformation takes time. If your trainer-candidate identifies appearance change as an intended outcome it ought to be mentioned in a demure tone with the clear message it will take time.

What to watch out for:

- *Guaranteeing radical body transformation*
(Some) Body transformation will occur if protocol is followed to foster health-related fitness gains, but without augmentation it is wholly unrealistic to suggest (then expect) that radical transformation will occur. We simply are genetically predisposed to certain realities—short torso, long arms, narrow shoulders—of which no amount of cardio or weight training will transform. Guaranteeing that transformation can occur that trumps genetics is absurd, but unfortunately prevalent.

- Guaranteeing that transformation will occur quickly, or within a certain time frame
While transformation can occur as a result of engaging in physical activity, it bears repeating—change appears over time, never overnight. In fact, change is first felt, and then appearance changes are noticed. Upon adherence to an achievement-oriented fitness routine we notice we feel stronger (cardiovascular and muscular) before we detect appearance changes. It simply takes time for transformation to occur, and the timeframe is unique to each of us. To suggest transformation will occur quickly or even within a certain timeframe is irresponsible, risks eroding motivation, and indicates gross incompetence.

  If claims about results seem outrageous then no doubt they are.

Do you keep a record of training sessions?

What to look for:

- *Clear indication/confirmation that the trainer-candidate keeps a record of each delivered training session*
Learning, in the form of health-related fitness gain, requires time and will occur if training sessions are purposeful, intentional, and progressive. Assessment and planning

cannot be left to chance. Maintaining records of your current levels of performance ensures that the demand at which you are working is appropriate. Maintaining records of training sessions ensures alignment from one session to the next and prevents undue repetition. Competent trainer-candidates understand that maintaining written records is as an important professional obligation.

What to watch out for:

* *Eschewing the importance of keeping records, underscored by a cavalier stance that record keeping is unnecessary*
  No matter how much content knowledge a trainer-candidate possesses, training need to be based upon accurate assessment of your performance levels and aligned from one session to the next. Written records ensure this information is captured. Without this information it is much less likely that your training experience will be purposeful or aligned one session to the next. This makes it much less likely that you will fully reap health-related benefits. Haphazardly planned training sessions lead to haphazard outcomes.

  Further, without a plan, it can be easy for trainers to lose sight of your level of performance, and thus not offer appropriate accommodation for the gains you make. This is of particular importance because with exercise, over time our body adapts to the stress put upon it. Continued improvement is contingent upon making adjustments to our routines to account for our gains in strength, endurance, or range of motion; all the more making the point that the routine in which we engage has to be planned. It is perfectly normal to hit performance plateaus. But appropriate adjustments made to your routine will prevent unnecessary plateauing, which can be frustrating and lead to diminished motivation. Your trainer ought to have a clearly articulated, written plan to guide your progress.

Do you engage in professional development? If so, what?

What to look for:

- *Evidence of regular, ongoing, consistent attendance at conferences, seminars, workshops, or coursework BEYOND what is required for certification renewal*
  Research that informs our understanding of health-related fitness is ongoing. The results of this research are disseminated through various means—for example, presentations at conferences, seminars and workshops, and written articles for professional journals. Keeping in mind that content knowledge is that which distinguishes a quality trainer from an ineffective one, it is imperative that a trainer stays current.

- *Evidence of sustained membership in professional organizations—AAHPERD, I.D.E.A. for example*
  Belonging to a professional organization indicates dedicated commitment to one's profession as a trainer. For one, it affords networking opportunities with other like-minded fitness professionals. It also requires an out-of-pocket expense, so the willingness to pay points to one's regard for his/her's professional status.

- *Evidence of regularly and consistently reading research*
  The disciplines and sub-disciplines aligned to health-related fitness have active, robust research communities. These efforts are constantly helping us understand the nuances of attaining and sustaining the health-protective benefits of physical activity participation. Numerous professional journals exist that publish the results of the conducted research. These results arm trainers with up-to-date information about effective training protocol, including that relating to safety.

What to watch out for:

- *No formal, ongoing professional development activity*

No matter the degree of talent one possesses to be a quality trainer, lack of formal, ongoing professional development will stagnate anyone's capacity.

- *Dismissing the necessity for ongoing professional development*
  The conduct of personal training lends itself to developing a consistent, rhythmic routine—clients are seen every hour beginning at the top of the hour and during that hour engage in a similar flow of activity from one client to the next. Developing a work routine is not unique to personal training, but the sense of routine is all the more pronounced since the routines trainers establish for themselves are comprised of the routines they conduct with their clientele. Therefore, it can be easy for trainers to fall into a flow where beginnings and endings get skewed. Additionally, physical activity professionals tend to establish professional behavior that is very stable—that is, they deliver instruction and provide feedback similarly from one client/class to the next. Without consistent, ongoing professional development to inform and offer insight about one's conduct, the routine can become *all too* routine. At stake is professional stagnation which can lend itself to fostering diminished achievement with clients.

  Further, the ongoing flow of research continues to inform our understanding of physical activity's bearing on health and wellness and prompts awareness of current health-related trends. A trainer's professional development habit can help ensure that your engagement is in line with up-to-date protocol for how to best sustain the benefits that activity participation can yield.

Do you possess the ability to foster motor-skill development (catching, throwing, kicking, striking, etc.)?

What to look for:

- *"Yes. This is an important part of your physical self, so we will work on your motor skills."*

- *"I can try so I can further help foster your physical self."*
  This is an honest response that conveys his/her interest in helping you reach your physical best and implies the trainer would do his/her best to facilitate the process of fostering your motor skills.

What to watch out for:

- *"No—why would you ask?"*
  This response indicates both a lack of content knowledge and professional demeanor. Motor-skill development mitigates our ability and motivation to engage in physical activity outside of the realm of fitness-based exercise. Playing basketball or softball, for example, whether in leagues or pick-up games, offers additional opportunities to foster the health benefits that can be yielded from physical activity participation. But, it simply isn't realistic to consider taking part in an activity requiring certain motor skill proficiency if one's skills are under-developed. Any personal trainer ought to promote engaging in as much physical activity as possible and possess the capacity to hone motor skills. It's likely that one whose professional preparation consisted of a short-term, superficial (i.e., weekend) program possesses neither the knowledge, inclination, nor understanding to address motor-skill development. One whose preparation was based upon a college degree in kinesiology, physical education, exercise science, or the like ought to well understand the importance of motor skill development and possess the pedagogical knowledge to foster improvement.

Note: The above questions provide a frame from which you can ascertain your trainer-candidate's professional capacity. The responses can help you determine his/her content knowledge, scope of experience, attitude toward working with someone of your age/gender, and degree of commitment to the training profession. As your conversation transpires there are also other dynamics/themes to pay attention to:

Hesitancy in responses

Sometimes pauses are necessary for one to gather his/her thoughts. If a pause is used as such then likely the responses will have meaning. But if the responses following pauses offer no insight, this indicates that the content knowledge is as well.

Defensiveness

Defensive responses or an overall defensive demeanor during the process speaks for itself. A quality trainer is one with the approach of "there you are" not "here I am." *Emphasis on appearance (rather than) performance goals/outcomes, or body transformations to acquire the body shape of someone else*

None of us can look like anyone but ourselves. To covertly or overtly suggest that appearance goals trump other goals undermines the most important aspect of training— providing health protection. Your health-related fitness potential will be sorely compromised if your trainer seeks results that are at all related to acquiring the body shape of someone else. While the suggestion is absurd and disturbing, the suggestion persists.

Unrealistic/dangerous promises about outcomes

Promising body transformation is dangerous for how it impacts the intent of the process and motivation. Promising transformation in a short period of time, i.e., two weeks, can be health threatening. If a suggestion seems outrageous and unrealistic then it likely is both.

Reference to the process being easy

Health-related fitness benefits (health protection) are the result of regular, appropriate physical activity participation (meaning abiding by the principles that guide health-related achievement). No ifs, ands, or buts. Insinuating the process is easy is simply wrong and misleading and can profoundly erode motivation. Hard work doesn't have to be equated with unpleasantness, though. And when through regular, appropriate physical activity participation you begin to feel and see results, your motivation to sustain your routine will be strengthened.

Step Two: Participate In A Trial Training Session With Your Trainer-Candidate and Assess His/Her Professional Conduct Accordingly

Immediately following your trial training session, reflect upon the following. You may want to jot down notes, as the process of writing your responses can all the more help you capture the experience (and ultimately judge the professional capacity of the trainer-candidate and determine if you want to offer employment).

Did your trainer-candidate...

- *Inquire about your general health and any activity limitations you might have prior to beginning the training session? Use a systematic process to assess your current level of fitness?*

  Safety is rule number one. Seeking information about any conditions or limitations a trainee presents is essential to ensuring that the training protocol is safe. Assessing current level of fitness ought to be conducted prior to engaging in activity. Most fitness facilities adopt and use an assessment tool to ascertain this information. It is expected that your trainer-candidate would use this assessment tool

- *Explain why each activity was being done?*

  An achievement-oriented health-related fitness routine is characterized by the feature of *purpose*, and the critical purpose is your physical well-being, which is comprised of the components of health-related fitness. It follows that each activity/exercise performed ought to address a health-related fitness component. Also, our motivation to engage in exercise is enhanced by knowing its purpose. Last, quality trainers share information to educate their clients. Health-related fitness is not proprietary to trainers.

- *Mention the components of health-related fitness? And comfortably explain/talk about each in a conversational manner? And use examples that you understood?*

  Those who have the capacity to deliver results will ensure that each and every activity done is purposeful toward a health-related fitness benefit. Regardless of the session being a trial, the trainer-candidate ought to have had you engaging in purposeful activities, NOT taking in a buffet of machines and seemingly touring the facility. Related, quality physical activity professionals are able to communicate health-related fitness achievement principles effortlessly and use specific examples to clarify/illustrate their description. Those whose preparation has been deficient are unable to do so clearly, specifically, or in an easy-to-understand manner. Not being able to converse about these concepts in a conversational manner is evidence that they themselves do not clearly understand them.

- *Use anatomically correct/appropriate language when describing the physiology and/or musculature of activities? Not "tummy," for example?*

  We are who we are—anatomy is anatomy. Using euphemisms to label body parts indicates a certain level of professional discomfort—perhaps a lack of vocabulary, an issue owning one's presence as a leader, or feeling the need to dumb-down. Note: it is much more likely trainer-candidates use passive, whimsical euphemisms with females than male clients. The ability to accurately yet casually speak about concepts helps ensure understanding, but using nonprofessional or dumbed-down language reflects a lack of credibility, and trivializes the experience.

- *Use gender-free language and project a gender-free attitude regarding physical activity participation? For example, no "boy" or "girl" push-ups or reference to machines being gender-specific?*

Genderized language is an indication of discriminatory practice. Certain physical activities can be MODIFIED to promote success and achievement (e.g., push-ups on your knees rather than arms), but modification is gender-neutral. Resistance machines and equipment also are not genderized. The flat bench press bench is not for men only, nor is the hip abduction machine for women only.

- *Call you by your first or last name?*

Using "sweetie" or "hon" or "sweatheart" or similar is simply unacceptable. While it may be wholly unintended, these terms are disrespectful and demeaning. One, it is highly doubtful that a trainer-candidate would refer to a male client using these terms. Two, it implies an unbal-anced relationship between the two of you—the trainer-candidate eliciting more power.

- *Encourage and promote full-body resistance training rather than gender discriminating by focusing upon purported "trouble spots" such as buttocks, hips, underarm jiggle?*

Muscular strength and endurance is each a component of health-related fitness. Achieving in both of these realms requires a program that hits all the major muscle groups. Focusing on eliminating or reducing a "weakness" with-out consideration to full-body conditioning will yield un-derachievement. Spot reduction simply is not possible! Developing robust physical wellness requires total-body conditioning.

- *Provide **specific** corrective or performance-related feedback? For example, that related to your lifting technique or movement gait, as well as motivational prompts and encouragement–e.g., "good job," "you can do it?"*

For reasons of safety and achievement, the movement we execute needs to be carefully monitored. Doing any exercise incorrectly, even a slight deviation from a safe angle of movement, can lead to injury. It will also lead to underachievement. Therefore, your trainer needs to consistently provide specific, corrective, performance-related feedback related to each exercise you perform when necessary. This includes your positioning on equipment. Weight machines tend to dwarf smaller-framed exercisers, typically women. This can put users in biomechanically dangerous lifting positions unless modifications (e.g., pads) are utilized. As well, users need to stand up straight when on the treadmill or elliptical. Feedback related to positioning on equipment needs to be as specific/corrective as that related to the movement itself.

A lack of this kind of feedback indicates complacency or one who simply doesn't have the professional capacity to know any better, neither serving your best interest.

Motivational prompts such as "good job" or "keep going" can help sustain effort but do nothing to inform us of our performance. Trainer-candidates who fail to provide specific, performance-related, or corrective feedback likely lack content knowledge (are not familiar with the nuances of a specific exercise movement) and/or an awareness of how important this is to the training process. Neither is conducive to delivering health-related fitness results.

Similarly, hustles and prompts may incite a trainee to work TOO hard—or at a greater intensity than is appropriate to their age or performance level. As much as not working hard enough compromises reaping the health-related benefits that can be derived, working too hard can be dangerous. Depending on age and any other health-related mitigating factors, intensity or heart rate needs to stay at or under what is recommended. Prompting effort that results in a heart rate that exceeds the recommendation is wholly inexcusable.

Further, trainers ought to approach clients from a teaching rather than a coaching perspective. (No disrespect to coaches.) The distinction here is how the power in the relationship transpires. Trainers ought to be of the mindset and practice that a shared partnership exists between them and their clients. Communication ought to emanate from an interest in conveying information rather than dictating orders.

- *Indicate what would comprise subsequent sessions and explain the need to modify the training protocol regularly to avoid plateaus or diminished results?*

Our bodies are remarkable for their ability to adapt to the stresses placed upon them. If regular modifications are not made to our training protocol we likely will plateau. Over time, doing the same exercises over and over utilizing the same intensity, effort, or resistance will result in diminished results. Upon adaptation, what initially stimulated results no longer will. Effective trainers understand the concept of "periodization" and know that modifications to one's routine need to be regularly infused (every ten to twelve weeks).

- *Focus on and reiterate the health-related fitness gains each exercise or exercise cluster would address? And NOT mention the potential changes to appearance that the exercises could potentially invoke?*

Health-related fitness change occurs from the inside out— training certainly can change your physique, but the initial changes occur at the cellular level. Each time you engage in physical activity according to the principles that guide health-related fitness, you will experience benefit—i.e., endorphin release, improved blood flow. Over time you will experience additional benefit—i.e, improved blood pressure, improved stroke volume, improved muscular strength. The initial benefit isn't what you can see, rather what is occurring within, such as a stronger cardiovascular system and how you feel during tasks such as being able to more easily carry your groceries. Over time you will begin to notice changes to your physique such as more musculature and a more defined musculature.

The point here is that your trainer-candidate ought to describe the health-related gains you can realize by doing certain exercises rather than referencing the physique or appearance changes that are possible. After all, health protection ought to frame our ultimate purpose for exercising.

• *Shift power to you—the one served—and offer information and strategies about exercising and self-monitoring?*

Just today, I overheard a trainer lament to a new client about the new client's financial reality of being able to work with the trainer twice a month. The (obnoxious) trainer made it clear that he saw clients at least twice a week, most more often, which of course wasn't something the new client didn't already know. The client's body language showed defeat—already she had failed. Sad to witness!

For the short term of your process together, your trainer ought to own the process of teaching, monitoring, and motivating you to develop and maintain an achievement-oriented health-related fitness routine. For the long term, though, your wellness is yours to sustain. At some point, actually beginning from the get-go, your trainer ought to shift the responsibility of your health-related fitness to you. Yes, separation ought to occur! This isn't to say that once separated you should not seek periodic tune-ups or check-ins, but your health-related fitness is about you—it is not about your trainer. Don't let it become about your trainer and don't fall prey to your trainer making it about him/her. The process is not about you making your trainer happy. Rather it's about you optimizing your health-related fitness. Effective trainers foster results, but at the same time share power with their clients.

- *Devote his/her full attention to you? For example, no phone calls, texts, wandering conversations, etc.?*

  Perhaps speaking for itself, this point seems blatantly unnecessary to mention. But it needs to be reiterated that your work with your trainer needs to be about you. It isn't the time for the trainer-candidate to chat up other exercisers or take or make phone calls or text messages. Of course some common sense here—exchanging quick hellos as other exercisers pass by is certainly fine. In fact, if your trainer-candidate is simply unfriendly or unresponsive to passing exchanges that is a red flag.

- *Ask your trainer-candidate for a reference*, specifically someone similar to you—gender, age, fitness level.

  Use the reference to further ascertain the trainer-candidate's consistency—between what s/he says s/he does and actually does, and ability to foster achievement—what health-related gains have been made? Toward both, also ask the reference if anything unexpected has occurred during training sessions, and if so how it was handled. Last, use the reference to source any particulars that a new client ought to be aware of.

  Competent service providers understand that professional reputation is earned through the relationships developed with clients. If your trainer-candidate is unwilling or unable to provide a reference it indicates, for example, a lack of confidence in his/her capacity, uncertainty about his/her standing with clients, and not regarding the work seriously; all symptoms of professional incompetency.

Additional Red Flags to Consider:

If your trainer-candidate:

- Encouraged "toning" or "shaping"

- • Guaranteed that body shape can be profoundly modified to look like…
- • Spoke of "spot reducing"
- • Spoke of an "easy" way/method/strategy or gimmick to achieve fitness results
- • Spoke of "THE best diet" to adopt or faddish ones promising (unrealistic, unsafe) fast results
- • Seemed to dumb-down the language used to communicate the exercise activities or the expectation for achievement itself
- • Used "just" to describe exercises or expected outcomes

Without hesitation, seek another trainer-candidate. The mention of any of these indicates sorely deficient professional capacity. This is not who you or anyone wants as their personal trainer. He/she will not be able to deliver health-related fitness results and you will under-realize the benefits of physical activity engagement. In fact, should you choose to, this information would be useful to the gym facility's management staff, especially to whoever oversees the personal training cadre.

Group Fitness Leaders and Small-Group Personal Trainers

A brief addition to the discussion of personal training competence is assessing the professional competence of a group fitness leader or a trainer who conducts group training sessions.

We have all been in group exercise classes lead by those considered great and other classes by those considered poor. One reality of group fitness is that participants will not return if they don't feel the leader is good. Who knew BODYPUMP or Pilates or spinning could be such cold, hard, cutthroat environments!

Primarily due to financial constraints, many gym-goers seek small group personal training (three to four clients at once) rather than one-on-one training. This can be a useful solution to an economic issue and when appropriately structured and delivered by a competent trainer, can yield the same health-related fitness achievement as one-on-one training.

Group fitness trends have been and likely will continue to be established by uber-charismatic personalities, but take care to assess your class leader for the professional competency he/she possesses, not just their fun personality. Charisma can make for an uplifting, joyous, and festive sixty minutes but the experience has to be deeper to foster your health protection. Similarly, training as part of a small group can offer the aspect of socialization and distraction unlike one-on-one training, but sessions need to be focused upon achievement.

Group fitness leaders and small-group trainers need to possess the professional competency to account for the diverse developmental differences present in any group fitness class or small-group training clientele.

Success has to be ensured for *each* group fitness class participant or each small-group training member. Therefore, leaders/trainers need to possess the knowledge and ability to offer modifications accordingly.

A primary question for you to consider if you take group classes or train with a small group: Does the leader/trainer help ME realize success?

If so, terrific! If not, try another one or another…

Points to Consider Once You Have Established a Relationship With a Personal Trainer, or if you are already working with a trainer

Assessing your trainer's professional competency doesn't end once you have agreed to a contract. Like changing the oil in your car, you need to conduct regular check-ups to ensure your trainer is fostering achievement, or otherwise an accountable partner to your health-related well-being. Whether it's a new trainer you selected by using the suggested protocol or one you were already working with, every 3-4 months you ought to ask yourself:

- **Are my muscles stronger?**
- **Have I built more muscle mass?**
- **Has my cardiovascular endurance improved/ strengthened?**
- **Do I have greater range-of-motion?**
- **Have I learned anything about fitness (from my trainer)?**
- **Am I (more) motivated to engage in physical activity?**
- **Has my body composition improved?**
- **Have markers of wellness improved?**

In addition, reflect upon the routines s/he prescribes and consider:

- Are the routines repetitious?
  The components of health-related fitness are fixed, but what is done to foster their achievement ought to regularly change. Variety is the spice of life, and the gym. The manner in which we work toward health-related achievement is limited only by the creativity of the one guiding the work. Creativity often comes persistent reflection, as in taking the time to conjure the gazillion ways one can have their client move to foster achievement. The same can become boring fast, but more important yields diminishing achievement, also fast. If the routine your trainer prescribes guides becomes routine, s/he simply isn't prepared to guide your achievement.

- Does my trainer copy what other trainers do?
  The gym is a very public milieu. While we all get caught up into our own routines, don't think for a second what we do doesn't go unnoticed by others. If but for a moment, what we do gets noticed by someone else. This can be the same for trainers. In some ways this isn't necessarily a

negative, for sharing among professionals certainly can enhance professional development. Unfortunately, the sharing process doesn't always stem from such good intent. For reasons like lack of planning, an underdeveloped activity repertoire, or limited content knowledge, trainers copy what they see other trainers doing without really having a clue why the exercise is being done or its safety considerations. Leading to, you guessed it, your underachievement.

For example, two current, 'trendy' gym routine components illustrate how copying can be problematic. The first is bench step-ups. Bench step-ups involve using some sort of a raised platform to step up on. Done correctly, bench step-ups can be yield cardiovascular and muscular benefit. The exercise certainly can get one's heart rate into its target zone, and foster total leg strengthening. The problem is trainers selecting a platform that is either too tall (high) or too short (low) for their client. Usually due to availability or proximity, the benches used for free weights are those used for step-ups. For the vast majority of women (comparatively shorter than men), these benches are too tall (high), requiring a severe, steep knee angle to complete the step-up. This movement stresses the hip, knee, and ankle joints unduly. Done at the correct height, bench step-ups are effective; done incorrectly they are dangerous!

The second is using a flight of stairs as the basis for cardio or leg work. Like bench step-ups, running stairs certainly can yield cardiovascular and muscular benefit. But too often it is prescribed with limited direction and lack of clear purpose. Doing "10 times up and down" may or may not yield cardio benefit. Most likely only a limited benefit as the prescribed "10" is either too many or too few considering one's fitness level, thus neither the duration of the exercise nor level of intensity is appropriate to yield optimum benefit. As well, bounding up and down can stress joints, especially if the rise of the stairs is not compatible to one's height (leg length). The knee angle created as one reaches up for the next step commonly is too steep, thus compromising joint safety.

Prescribing bench step-ups or stair running after seeing other trainers do it with their clients can be useful IF either's purpose and safety is ensured. Otherwise, both not only will yield limited benefit, but will be dangerous!

In general, and barring complication, 3-4 months is a reasonable timeframe in which to expect results (improvement), (and subsequently every 3-4 months thereafter). The answers to these questions will make a clear case for either continuing to work with your trainer, or reviewing Steps 1 and 2 of "Assessing the Professional Competency of Your Personal Trainer" and initiating project find-a new-trainer.

Don't over think the process; don't make excuses; but most important, don't enable your trainer's underachievement. Use the information you gather to objectively determine if your trainer deserves to remain your trainer.

Final Farewell

So we have come to the end, and just like a quality training session ending with a warm-down this too is the time to reflect, and with renewed vim take stock of just who is minding your store. And, you are ready—ready to realize optimum health-related achievement by ensuring that your trainer can deliver. You know what to ask, you know what to look for and you know what to do. I assure you there is a good personal trainer waiting for you RIGHT NOW.

Always remember that the stakes are simply too high to leave your fitness to chance. Being a well intended but mis-informed or under-informed fitness professional is not good enough. Don't ever compromise your well-being by working with (and paying!) a trainer who does not possess the attitude or aptitude to be accountable to your health-related achievement. His or her underachievement should not yield your underachievement.

Look for me at the gym. I'll be the sweaty smiling one happy to see you working with a trainer who works as hard as you toward your well-being.

My best to you for prosperous health!

Bibliography

American College of Sports Medicine, Barbara Bushman, (Ed.) (2011). *ACSM's complete guide to fitness and health*. Human Kinetics.

American Heart Association. http://www.heart.org

Berg, K. (2011). *Prescriptive stretching*. Human Kinetics.

Centers for Disease Control and Prevention (CDC). http://www.cdc.gov

Cissik, J. (2005). *The basics of strength training*. Macgraw-Hill.

Fahey, T. (2009). *Basic weight training for men and women*. Macgraw-Hill.

Fleck, S. & Kraemer, W. (2004). *Designing resistance training programs-3rd edition*. Human Kinetics

National Institute of Health. http://www.nih.gov.

Sharkey, B. & Gaskill, S. (2007). *Fitness & health-6th edition*. Human Kinetics.

Silverman, S. & Ennis, C. (Eds.) ( ). *Student learning in physical education*. Human Kinetics.

Sandler, D. (2010). *Fundamental weight training*. Human Kinetics.

Appendix A: NCCA-accredited Personal Training Organizations

(International Health, Racquet and Sportsclub Association, as of February, 2011)

- Academy of Applied Personal Training Education (AAPTE), www.aapte.org
- American College of Sports Medicine (ACSM), www.acsm.org
- American Council on Exercise (ACE), www.acefitness.org
- Cooper Institute, www.cooperinstitute.org
- International Fitness Professionals Association (IFPA), www.ifpa-fitness.com
- National Academy of Sports Medicine (NASM), www.nasm.org
- National Council on Strength and Fitness (NCSF), www.ncsf.org
- National Exercise and Sports Trainers Association (NESTA), www.nestacertified.com
- National Exercise Trainers Association (NETA), www.netafit.org
- National Federation of Professional Trainers (NFPT), www.nfpt.com
- National Strength and Conditioning Association (NSCA), www.nsca-lift.org
- Training and Wellness Certification Commission (TWCC), www.personaltrainer.com

ENDNOTES

1   * It bears repeating: not all physical activity participation is the same. Whereas any physical activity is better than no physical activity, underachievement—less health protection, less health-related fitness—will occur if we do not engage in activity according to the principles known to elicit benefit.

2   *American Heart Association. (2011, December) *New stats show America's heart health need improvement.* Retrieved January 16, 2012, from
     http://newsroom.heart.org/pr/aha/new-stats-show-america-s-heart-220506.aspx

3   * Proctor, D., Melton, L., Khosla, S., Crowson, C., O'Conner, M. & Riggs, B. (2000). Relative influence of physical activity, muscle mass and strength on bone density. *Osteoporosis International,* 11 (11), 944-952.

4   * Retrieved July 2, 2011 from http://www.chiropractor-finder. com/great-reasons-for-visiting-chiropractors.html

5   * Reiteration of having earned a *reputable* fitness certification that addresses health-related fitness and assesses a prospective trainer's understanding of the content: knowing that content knowledge is THE primary factor that separates the best from the okay, it would be prudent to ascertain the certification requirements that your prospective trainer completed. He/she ought to be able to comfortably and concisely speak about the components included in the preparation program. You can prompt about content knowledge specific to health-related fitness, but prompts really should not be necessary because communicating the principles ought to be the primary focus of any trainer candidate. It would be a red flag if you find you have to prompt to ascertain

your candidate's grasp of content knowledge. There are solid preparation programs and there are lousy ones. Take the time to listen to your trainer-candidate, always from the perspective of protecting your health-related fitness. The tone and content of his/her response regarding professional preparation will tell you all you need to know.

www.ingramcontent.com/pod-product-compliance
Lightning Source LLC
Chambersburg PA
CBHW060209290526
45789CB00003B/1217